Red Light Therapy for Beginners

The Science Behind Red Light Therapy

By

Callum Bryden

Table of Contents

CHAPTER 1 4

Introduction 4

1.1 What is Red Light Therapy? 5

1.2 Benefits of Red-Light Therapy 6

CHAPTER 2 11

Understanding Red Light Therapy ..11

2.1 The Science Behind Red Light Therapy.................................... 12

2.2 Different Types of Light Therapy..................................... 15

2.3 How Does Red Light Therapy Work? 17

CHAPTER 3 20

Choosing the Right Red-Light Device 20

3.1 Factors to Consider................. 20

3.2 Types of Red-Light Devices ..24

CHAPTER 4 28

Getting Started.............................28

4.1 Preparing for Your Red-Light
Therapy Session 28

4.2 Safety Precautions 32

4.3 Setting Up Your Red-Light
Device...35

CHAPTER 5 42

Using Red Light Therapy for Health
and Wellness.................................42

5.1 Skin Health and Beauty..........42

5.2 Pain Relief and Inflammation 46

5.3 Muscle Recovery and Athletic
Performance 49

5.4 Sleep Improvement 51

5.5 Mood and Mental Health........54

CHAPTER 6.................................58

Tips for Success...........................58

6.1 Frequency and Duration of
Sessions 58

6.2 Maximizing Benefits 63

6.3 Tracking Your Progress 68

6.4 Next Steps in Your Red-Light
Therapy Journey 74

CHAPTER 1
Introduction

Red Light Therapy, also known as Low-Level Light Therapy (LLLT) or photobiomodulation, is a non-invasive therapeutic technique that utilizes red and near-infrared light to improve a variety of health and wellness-related conditions. It has gained popularity in recent years due to its potential benefits and its minimal side effects, making it an attractive option for individuals seeking alternative or complementary approaches to healthcare.

1.1 What is Red Light Therapy?

Red Light Therapy involves the use of low-energy, red or near-infrared light wavelengths to penetrate the skin and interact with cells in the body. These wavelengths typically range from approximately 630 to 850 nanometers and are in the non-ionizing radiation spectrum, which means they do not have the harmful properties associated with ultraviolet (UV) rays.

The key principle behind Red Light Therapy is photobiomodulation, which refers to the process where light energy is absorbed by cellular components, leading to various biological effects. It stimulates cellular energy production, specifically in the form of adenosine triphosphate (ATP), the cell's energy currency. This increase in energy production promotes several positive changes within the body.

Red Light Therapy can be administered through a variety of devices, including low-level laser therapy (LLLT) devices, light-emitting diode (LED) panels, and handheld units. These devices emit red and near-infrared light, which is applied directly to the skin or tissues in the targeted area. The therapy is non-thermal, meaning it doesn't produce heat, and is considered safe for most individuals.

1.2 Benefits of Red-Light Therapy

Red Light Therapy offers a wide range of potential benefits, and its applications continue to expand as research in the field grows. Some of the key benefits and therapeutic applications of Red Light Therapy include:

1. Improved Skin Health: Red Light Therapy can help with various skin conditions such as acne, wrinkles, scars, and age spots. It stimulates the production of collagen and elastin, leading to smoother, more youthful-looking skin.

2. Pain Relief and Inflammation Reduction: Red Light Therapy has been used to alleviate pain and reduce inflammation in conditions such as arthritis, joint pain, and muscle injuries. It may help by increasing blood flow and promoting the release of endorphins, the body's natural painkillers.

3. Enhanced Muscle Recovery and Athletic Performance: Many athletes and fitness enthusiasts use Red Light Therapy to speed up muscle recovery after intense workouts and improve their overall performance. The therapy can reduce muscle fatigue and the risk of injury.

4. Wound Healing: Red Light Therapy may accelerate the healing of wounds, cuts, and surgical incisions. It does so by increasing cell proliferation and improving circulation, which can aid in tissue repair.

5. Improved Sleep: Some individuals report better sleep quality and reduced insomnia symptoms after using Red Light Therapy. By positively affecting circadian rhythms and promoting relaxation, it can help regulate sleep patterns.

6. Mood and Mental Health: Red Light Therapy is being investigated for its potential to alleviate symptoms of depression and anxiety. It may do so by influencing neurotransmitter levels in the brain and improving overall mental well-being.

7. Hair Growth: Red Light Therapy has shown promise in stimulating hair follicles, potentially leading to increased hair growth and reduced hair loss in conditions like androgenetic alopecia.

It's important to note that the effectiveness of Red-Light Therapy can vary among individuals and may depend on factors such as the specific condition being treated, the wavelength and dosage of light used, and the consistency of therapy. While many people experience positive outcomes, individual responses may differ.

Red Light Therapy is a versatile and non-invasive approach to health and wellness that harnesses the power of red and near-infrared light to stimulate cellular processes and provide various benefits. Its potential applications continue to expand, making it an intriguing option for those seeking alternatives or complementary therapies to improve their overall well-being. As with any medical or wellness intervention, it's advisable to consult with a healthcare professional before beginning Red Light Therapy to ensure it's suitable for your specific needs and conditions.

CHAPTER 2

Understanding Red Light Therapy

Red Light Therapy is a fascinating field that bridges science and health and has the potential to offer a wide range of therapeutic benefits. To appreciate its applications fully, it's essential to understand the science behind it, the different types of light therapy available, and the mechanisms through which Red Light Therapy exerts its effects.

2.1 The Science Behind Red Light Therapy

Red Light Therapy is grounded in the science of photobiomodulation. At its core, this therapy leverages the unique properties of red and near-infrared light to interact with biological systems on a cellular level. The key principles involved in the science of Red Light Therapy are as follows:

- **Photon Absorption:** When red or near-infrared light is applied to the skin, photons are absorbed by chromophores within the cells, with cytochrome c oxidase being a significant target. This absorption of photons stimulates a series of photochemical reactions in the mitochondria of the cell.

- **Enhanced ATP Production:**
  The energy derived from these
  reactions results in an increase
  in adenosine triphosphate
  (ATP) production. ATP is the
  molecule responsible for
  storing and transporting energy
  within cells, and higher levels
  of ATP have a profound impact
  on cellular function.

- **Cellular Effects:** The increased
  ATP production influences
  various cellular processes,
  including improved DNA
  synthesis, cell proliferation, and
  the release of signaling
  molecules. This, in turn, leads
  to a cascade of biological
  effects that are responsible for
  the potential therapeutic
  benefits of Red Light Therapy.

- **Reduction of Oxidative Stress:** Red Light Therapy can reduce oxidative stress and inflammation by enhancing the activity of antioxidant enzymes and decreasing the production of harmful reactive oxygen species (ROS).

- **Gene Expression and Protein Synthesis:** The therapy can also influence gene expression and protein synthesis, which can result in changes in cell behavior and function. This can be harnessed for various therapeutic purposes.

2.2 Different Types of Light Therapy

While Red Light Therapy is one of the most well-known forms of photobiomodulation, there are different types of light therapy that utilize various wavelengths and applications. These include:

- **Blue Light Therapy:** Used primarily to treat skin conditions, blue light therapy is effective against acne and other dermatological issues. It works by targeting and destroying the bacteria responsible for these skin conditions.

- **Green Light Therapy:** This therapy is often employed for skin pigmentation issues and to reduce redness. It has a calming effect on the skin and can help improve the appearance of certain skin conditions.

- **Yellow Light Therapy:** Yellow light therapy is used to reduce redness, swelling, and inflammation. It's often applied in conjunction with red light therapy for a more comprehensive approach to skin health.

- **Infrared Light Therapy:** This therapy utilizes infrared light, which penetrates deeper into the body than red light. Infrared light therapy is commonly used for pain relief, muscle recovery, and to stimulate the deeper tissues.

2.3 How Does Red Light Therapy Work?

The mechanisms through which Red Light Therapy works can be summarized as follows:

1. **Cellular Energy Boost:** Red and near-infrared light is absorbed by cells and stimulates the production of ATP, increasing cellular energy.

2. **Cellular Function Optimization:** This surplus energy enhances cellular functions, such as DNA synthesis, cell proliferation, and the release of signaling molecules.

3. **Tissue Repair and Healing:** Red Light Therapy can promote

tissue repair and wound healing by increasing blood flow, collagen production, and reducing inflammation.

4. **Pain Reduction:** By reducing inflammation and promoting tissue repair, Red Light Therapy can alleviate pain and discomfort in various conditions, including musculoskeletal pain.

5. **Mood and Sleep Regulation:** The therapy can positively affect mood and sleep patterns by influencing neurotransmitter levels and circadian rhythms.

In essence, Red Light Therapy works at a cellular level to improve the functioning of tissues, cells, and organs throughout the body. Its applications are diverse, from skin health to pain relief and mental well-being, making it an intriguing area of study and practice within the field of alternative and complementary medicine.

CHAPTER 3

Choosing the Right Red-Light Device

Selecting the right red light therapy device is a crucial step in ensuring you receive the maximum benefits from your therapy. To make an informed decision, you need to consider various factors and understand the different types of red-light devices available.

3.1 Factors to Consider

When choosing a red light therapy device, take the following factors into account:

1. **Wavelength and Spectrum:**
    Red light therapy typically
    involves red and near-infrared
    wavelengths. Different
    wavelengths may be more
    effective for specific
    applications, so ensure the
    device emits the appropriate
    spectrum for your intended use.

2. **Power and Irradiance:** The
    power of the device, often
    measured in milliwatts (mW) or
    watts (W), and irradiance,
    which is the power per unit area
    (mW/cm^2), determine the
    strength and depth of
    penetration. Consider the
    desired treatment area and the
    device's power output.

3. **Treatment Area:** Some
    devices are designed for small,
    localized treatment areas, while

others cover larger areas. Choose a device that suits the size of the area you plan to treat.

4. **Treatment Time:** Consider the recommended treatment time for your specific condition. Devices with higher irradiance may require shorter treatment sessions, which can be more convenient.

5. **Portability and Design:** Depending on your needs, you might prefer a portable or stationary device. Some devices are designed for home use, while others are more suitable for clinical or professional settings.

6. **Safety Features:** Look for devices that have safety

features, such as eye protection or automatic shutoff timers. Safety is a top priority when using any light therapy device.

7. **Ease of Use:** User-friendliness is important. Ensure the device is easy to operate and comes with clear instructions.

8. **FDA Approval:** Some devices have received FDA clearance for specific uses, which can provide additional confidence in their safety and efficacy.

9. **Price:** The cost of red light therapy devices varies widely. Set a budget and look for options that fit within it while still meeting your specific needs.

10. **Reviews and Recommendations:** Research

and read reviews from users who have used the device for similar purposes. Recommendations from healthcare professionals can also be valuable.

11. **Warranty and Customer Support:** Check the warranty and the level of customer support provided by the manufacturer. A good warranty can offer peace of mind, and reliable customer support can assist you with any questions or issues.

3.2 Types of Red-Light Devices

There are several types of red light therapy devices available:

1. **Handheld Devices:** These are
   small, portable devices that you
   can hold and use directly on the
   skin. They are suitable for
   localized treatments, such as
   facial skin care or targeting
   specific areas of pain.

2. **Panel Lights:** Panel lights are
   larger devices with multiple
   LED bulbs or diodes. They are
   designed to cover larger
   treatment areas and are often
   used for full-body therapy.

3. **Wearable Devices:** Some red
   light therapy devices are
   designed to be worn on the
   body, like a wrap or belt. These
   are ideal for hands-free
   treatments and can target
   specific areas.

4. **Combination Devices:** Some
   devices combine red light
   therapy with other therapies,
   such as infrared heat or
   ultrasound, for a
   comprehensive approach to
   wellness.

5. **Professional-Grade Devices:**
   These devices are typically
   found in clinical settings and
   offer higher power and
   versatility for more intensive
   therapy. They may require
   professional guidance.

Before purchasing a red-light therapy
device, carefully assess your needs
and the specific conditions you intend
to address. Consult with a healthcare
professional if you have any
uncertainties about which device is
best suited for your goals. Investing
the time to choose the right device

will ensure that you receive the
maximum benefits from your red light
therapy sessions.

CHAPTER 4

Getting Started

Before beginning your red-light therapy sessions, it's important to make preparations and understand the necessary safety precautions to ensure a safe and effective experience. Here's a guide on getting started with red light therapy:

4.1 Preparing for Your Red-Light Therapy Session

1. **Consult with a Healthcare Professional:** If you have any underlying medical conditions or are taking medications, it's a

good idea to consult with a healthcare professional before starting red light therapy. They can provide guidance on whether it's safe and appropriate for your specific situation.

2. **Choose the Right Device:** Ensure you have the appropriate red light therapy device for your needs, whether it's a handheld device, panel light, or wearable device. Check that the device is in good working condition, and follow the manufacturer's instructions for use.

3. **Set Up a Comfortable Space:** Find a quiet and comfortable space for your red light therapy sessions. Ensure you have

privacy and won't be disturbed during your treatment.

4. **Cleanse and Prepare the Skin:** If you're using red light therapy for skin health, make sure your skin is clean and free from lotions, creams, or makeup. Cleanse your skin gently before each session.

5. **Wear Appropriate Eye Protection:** Red light therapy devices emit intense light, and it's crucial to protect your eyes during the treatment. Use the provided eye protection or goggles that come with the device. Keep your eyes closed during the session, and do not look directly into the light source.

6. **Follow Recommended Dosage:** Pay attention to the recommended treatment time and dosage for your specific condition. Overusing the therapy or using it for longer than recommended does not necessarily yield better results and could potentially lead to adverse effects.

7. **Position Yourself Properly:** Position the device or yourself, if it's a handheld device, according to the instructions provided by the manufacturer. Maintain the recommended distance between the device and your skin for optimal results.

8. **Consistency is Key:** To achieve the desired results, be consistent with your red light

therapy sessions. It may take several weeks or months of regular use to see noticeable improvements, so establish a routine that works for you.

4.2 Safety Precautions

Red light therapy is generally considered safe, but it's essential to be aware of and follow safety precautions:

1. **Eye Protection:** Always wear the recommended eye protection to shield your eyes from the intense light emitted during the session. Direct exposure to the light can harm your eyes.

2. **Pregnancy:** If you are pregnant, consult with a

healthcare professional before using red light therapy, as its safety during pregnancy has not been extensively studied.

3. **Skin Sensitivity:** Some people may experience skin sensitivity or mild redness, especially during initial sessions. If this occurs, reduce the treatment time or distance from the device until your skin adapts.

4. **Photosensitivity:** If you are taking medications or using skincare products that make your skin more sensitive to light, consult with a healthcare professional before starting red light therapy.

5. **Limitation for Children:** Red light therapy is generally not recommended for children

unless under the guidance of a healthcare professional.

6. **Dosage Limits:** Avoid excessive exposure to red light therapy, as high doses may have adverse effects. Stick to the recommended treatment times and frequencies.

7. **Avoid Overheating:** If you're using a panel light or a device with a high wattage, be mindful of overheating. Ensure the room is well-ventilated and at a comfortable temperature.

8. **Hydration:** Drink plenty of water before and after your session, as increased cellular activity during red light therapy may lead to increased hydration needs.

By following these guidelines and safety precautions, you can make the most of your red-light therapy sessions while ensuring your well-being and safety. If you have any concerns or experience unusual reactions, discontinue the treatment and consult a healthcare professional.

4.3 Setting Up Your Red-Light Device

Setting up your red-light therapy device is a straightforward process, but it's important to follow the manufacturer's instructions carefully to ensure a safe and effective treatment. Here's a step-by-step guide to setting up your red-light device:

1. **Read the User Manual:** Start by thoroughly reading the user

manual or instructions provided by the manufacturer. The manual contains specific information about your device, including usage guidelines, recommended treatment times, and safety precautions.

2. **Choose a Suitable Location:** Find a quiet, private area where you can comfortably undergo your red-light therapy sessions. Ensure there are no distractions or interruptions during your treatment.

3. **Clean the Device:** If your device has been in storage, give it a quick wipe-down to remove any dust or debris. Make sure the lenses or light-emitting surfaces are clean and free from obstructions.

4. **Check the Power Source:**
    Ensure the device is properly
    connected to a reliable power
    source. Depending on your
    device, this could involve
    plugging it into an electrical
    outlet, inserting batteries, or
    charging it.

5. **Position the Device:** Set up the
    device according to the
    manufacturer's instructions.
    The exact positioning and
    distance from your skin may
    vary depending on the device
    type and the area you are
    targeting. Some devices require
    direct skin contact, while others
    are designed to be used at a
    specific distance. Follow the
    recommended guidelines for
    optimal results.

6. **Prepare Your Skin:** If you are using red light therapy for skin health, cleanse your skin gently to remove any makeup, lotions, or creams. Clean, dry skin enhances the effectiveness of the treatment.

7. **Put on Eye Protection:** Always wear the provided eye protection or goggles, as recommended by the manufacturer. Ensure your eyes are shielded from the intense light emitted during the session. Keep your eyes closed during the treatment.

8. **Power On the Device:** Turn on the red-light therapy device, following the manufacturer's instructions. Some devices may have different settings or wavelengths, so choose the

appropriate settings for your specific needs.

9. **Begin the Session:** Start your red light therapy session by placing the device or its light-emitting surface in the correct position. Activate the treatment according to the manufacturer's guidelines.

10. **Relax and Enjoy:** During the session, relax and enjoy the soothing and gentle warmth of the red light. You can read, meditate, or simply unwind while the therapy takes place.

11. **Monitor the Time:** Keep track of the recommended treatment time. Most sessions range from a few minutes to around 20 minutes, but it may vary

depending on your specific condition and device.

12. **Power Off and Store:** When the session is complete, turn off the device and follow any additional post-treatment instructions provided in the user manual. Properly store the device according to the manufacturer's recommendations.

13. **Clean and Maintain:** After each session, if necessary, clean the device as recommended in the user manual. Regular maintenance ensures the device remains in good working condition.

By following these steps, you can easily set up and use your red-light therapy device for safe and effective treatments. Consistency in following the recommended treatment guidelines is key to achieving the desired results. If you have any questions or concerns, don't hesitate to reach out to the device's manufacturer or consult with a healthcare professional.

CHAPTER 5

Using Red Light Therapy for Health and Wellness

Red Light Therapy is a versatile treatment with a wide range of applications in promoting health and wellness.

5.1 Skin Health and Beauty

Red Light Therapy has gained popularity in the field of skincare and beauty due to its potential to enhance the appearance and health of the skin.

Here's how it can be used for skin
health and beauty:

- **Collagen Production:** Red
  Light Therapy stimulates the
  production of collagen, a
  protein essential for
  maintaining skin's elasticity and
  youthful appearance. Collagen
  production can reduce the
  appearance of wrinkles, fine
  lines, and sagging skin.

- **Wound Healing:** Red Light
  Therapy promotes the healing
  of wounds, burns, and scars by
  accelerating cell growth and
  tissue repair. It can help reduce
  scarring and improve overall
  skin texture.

- **Acne Treatment:** Red Light
  Therapy can be effective in
  treating acne by reducing

inflammation and promoting healing. It targets the sebaceous glands, reducing excess oil production, and can also kill the bacteria responsible for acne.

- **Reduction of Hyperpigmentation:** For individuals with hyperpigmentation, red light therapy can help reduce the appearance of dark spots, sunspots, and other pigmentation issues by targeting melanin production.

- **Reduction of Redness and Rosacea:** Red light therapy can alleviate redness and symptoms associated with conditions like rosacea. It does so by reducing inflammation and promoting a healthier skin tone.

- **Hair Growth:** In addition to skin health, red light therapy has shown promise in stimulating hair growth. It may be used to treat conditions like androgenetic alopecia, promoting the growth of thicker and healthier hair.

To use red light therapy for skin health and beauty, it's important to follow a consistent treatment schedule, adhere to recommended treatment times and distances, and ensure your skin is clean and free from any substances that could block the light. Over time, with regular use, you may notice improvements in skin texture, tone, and overall appearance.

5.2 Pain Relief and Inflammation

Red Light Therapy has emerged as a promising approach for pain relief and the reduction of inflammation, both acute and chronic. Here's how it can be used in this context:

- **Muscle Recovery:** Athletes and individuals with muscle soreness or injuries often use red light therapy to speed up the recovery process. It can reduce muscle fatigue and promote faster healing.

- **Joint Pain and Arthritis:** Red Light Therapy has been shown to alleviate joint pain, whether due to conditions like arthritis or general wear and tear. It reduces inflammation and can improve joint mobility.

- **Back Pain:** Chronic back pain sufferers have reported relief from their symptoms through regular red light therapy sessions. The therapy can target specific areas of pain in the back, offering relief.

- **Injury Healing:** For various injuries, such as sprains, strains, or minor cuts, red light therapy can accelerate the healing process. It does this by increasing blood circulation and promoting tissue repair.

- **Reduction of Inflammation:** Red Light Therapy can help reduce inflammation in various parts of the body. This may be especially beneficial for individuals with chronic inflammatory conditions.

- **Pain Management:** Red Light Therapy may provide a non-invasive, drug-free option for pain management, allowing individuals to reduce their reliance on pain medications.

To use red light therapy for pain relief and inflammation, follow the recommended treatment guidelines for your specific condition. The frequency, duration, and power of the sessions may vary, so consult with a healthcare professional or the device manufacturer for guidance tailored to your needs. Red light therapy can be a valuable tool in managing pain and improving overall well-being.

5.3 Muscle Recovery and Athletic Performance

Red Light Therapy is increasingly recognized for its role in muscle recovery and enhancing athletic performance. Here's how it can benefit athletes and active individuals:

- **Faster Muscle Recovery:** Red Light Therapy promotes faster muscle recovery after intense workouts. It reduces muscle fatigue, inflammation, and oxidative stress, allowing athletes to return to training more quickly.

- **Reduced Muscle Soreness:** By decreasing muscle soreness and stiffness, red light therapy enables athletes to perform at their best, especially during high-intensity training periods.

- **Improved Endurance:** Enhanced cellular energy production from red light therapy can lead to improved endurance and overall athletic performance.

- **Reduced Risk of Injury:** By speeding up recovery and reducing inflammation, red light therapy can help lower the risk of exercise-related injuries.

- **Strength and Power Enhancement:** Some studies suggest that red light therapy may enhance strength and power output, making it valuable for athletes in strength sports.

To use red light therapy for muscle recovery and athletic performance, incorporate it into your post-workout routine. Apply the therapy to the muscles you've trained, following recommended treatment times and guidelines. Be consistent with your sessions to experience the full benefits.

5.4 Sleep Improvement

Red Light Therapy can also contribute to sleep improvement and regulation of circadian rhythms, offering potential benefits for those with sleep disturbances. Here's how it can be used to enhance sleep:

- **Circadian Rhythm Regulation:** Exposure to red light therapy in the morning can help regulate the body's internal clock (circadian rhythm). It may be particularly helpful for individuals with irregular sleep schedules, such as shift workers.

- **Melatonin Production:** Red Light Therapy has been shown to stimulate melatonin production, the hormone responsible for regulating sleep-wake cycles. Adequate melatonin levels are crucial for good sleep.

- **Reduction of Insomnia Symptoms:** Some individuals report reduced insomnia symptoms and improved sleep quality with regular red light therapy sessions, especially when used in the evening or before bedtime.

- **Mood and Relaxation:** Red Light Therapy may positively influence mood and promote relaxation, creating a more conducive environment for restful sleep.

To use red light therapy for sleep improvement, incorporate it into your daily routine. Light exposure in the morning or evening can help regulate your circadian rhythms. Be mindful of the timing and duration of your sessions, and aim for consistency to achieve the best results. If you have specific sleep disorders, consult with a healthcare professional for personalized guidance.

Red Light Therapy offers potential benefits for muscle recovery, athletic performance, and sleep improvement. Whether you're an athlete looking to enhance your training or an individual seeking better sleep, consider integrating red light therapy into your wellness routine while following recommended guidelines for optimal results.

5.5 Mood and Mental Health

Red Light Therapy is gaining attention for its potential to positively impact mood and mental health. While the field of photobiomodulation is still evolving in this area, there is evidence to suggest that red light therapy may have a range of effects that contribute to improved mental well-being. Here's how it can influence mood and mental health:

- **Neurotransmitter Activity:** Red Light Therapy has been shown to influence the activity of neurotransmitters in the brain, which play a crucial role in regulating mood. For example, it may enhance the release of serotonin, a neurotransmitter associated with feelings of well-being and happiness.

- **Stress Reduction:** Exposure to red light therapy may help reduce stress and anxiety levels. It can promote relaxation and decrease the production of stress hormones, such as cortisol.

- **Circadian Rhythm Regulation:** By influencing the body's internal clock (circadian rhythm), red light therapy can help establish healthier sleep-wake patterns, which can have a direct impact on mood and overall mental health.

- **Energy Levels:** Enhanced cellular energy production from red light therapy can lead to increased overall vitality, potentially reducing feelings of fatigue and enhancing mental alertness.

- **Seasonal Affective Disorder (SAD):** Some individuals with Seasonal Affective Disorder, a type of depression related to changes in seasons, may find relief from symptoms through exposure to red light therapy. Light therapy is a well-established treatment for SAD, and red light therapy could provide a more comfortable and convenient option.

- **Overall Well-Being:** The combined effects of improved sleep, reduced stress, and increased energy can contribute to an enhanced sense of well-being and improved mental health.

It's important to note that while there is evidence supporting these potential mental health benefits, the field of red light therapy in the context of mood and mental health is still emerging, and more research is needed to fully understand the mechanisms and best practices.

If you are considering using red light therapy to support your mood and mental health, consult with a healthcare professional to discuss your specific needs and circumstances. Additionally, ensure that you use the therapy as a complementary approach to other mental health strategies, such as therapy, exercise, and a balanced diet.

CHAPTER 6

Tips for Success

To achieve the best results with red light therapy, it's crucial to consider the frequency and duration of your sessions. These tips can help you make the most of your therapy:

6.1 Frequency and Duration of Sessions

1. **Consistency is Key:** Red light therapy is most effective when used consistently. Develop a regular schedule that you can adhere to. Whether it's daily, a few times a week, or weekly,

consistency is essential for optimal results.

2. **Adapt to Your Goals:** The frequency and duration of your sessions may vary depending on your specific goals. For general wellness, shorter, more frequent sessions may be suitable. For targeted conditions, longer sessions or higher frequency may be necessary.

3. **Start Slowly:** If you're new to red light therapy, begin with shorter sessions, especially for the first few weeks. This allows your body to adapt and reduces the risk of any adverse reactions.

4. **Consult a Healthcare Professional:** If you're using

red light therapy for a specific
medical condition or concern,
consult with a healthcare
professional. They can provide
guidance on the ideal frequency
and duration based on your
individual needs.

5. **Track Your Progress:** Keep a
   journal or record of your
   sessions, including the
   frequency and duration. This
   can help you track your
   progress over time and make
   adjustments if needed.

6. **Observe Your Body:** Pay
   attention to how your body
   responds to the therapy. Some
   individuals may experience
   benefits with shorter sessions,
   while others may need longer
   exposure. Adjust your approach
   based on your body's feedback.

7. **Increase Duration Gradually:**
    If you find that shorter sessions
    are not producing the desired
    results, you can gradually
    increase the duration. Start with
    a few additional minutes and
    monitor how your body
    responds.

8. **Prioritize Safety:** Be cautious
    not to overuse red light therapy.
    While it's generally considered
    safe, excessive exposure could
    lead to adverse effects. Follow
    the manufacturer's
    recommendations and consult
    with a healthcare professional if
    you have concerns.

9. **Set Realistic Expectations:**
    Red light therapy is not a quick
    fix, and results may take time.
    Set realistic expectations for

your specific goals and be patient with the process.

10. **Complement with Other Wellness Practices:** Red light therapy can be a valuable part of your wellness routine, but it's often most effective when combined with other healthy practices. This might include a balanced diet, regular exercise, and proper sleep.

The frequency and duration of red light therapy sessions can vary based on individual factors, the specific device used, and the desired outcomes. What works best for one person may not be suitable for another, so it's essential to customize your approach to align with your unique needs and goals.

6.2 Maximizing Benefits

To make the most of your red light therapy sessions and maximize the benefits, consider the following tips:

1. **Understand Your Goals:** Clearly define your objectives for using red light therapy. Whether it's skin health, pain relief, muscle recovery, or other specific goals, having a clear purpose will guide your treatment plan.

2. **Consult a Healthcare Professional:** If you have specific health concerns or conditions, consult with a healthcare professional or dermatologist before starting red light therapy. They can offer guidance tailored to your needs.

3. **Choose the Right Device:**
Select a high-quality red light
therapy device that suits your
goals and needs. Ensure it emits
the appropriate wavelengths
and power for your intended
use.

4. **Follow Manufacturer
Guidelines:** Adhere to the
manufacturer's instructions
regarding treatment times,
distances, and safety
precautions. These guidelines
are essential for safe and
effective therapy.

5. **Cleanse Your Skin:** Before
sessions targeting skin health or
beauty, ensure your skin is
clean and free from lotions,
makeup, or creams. Clean skin
enhances the therapy's
effectiveness.

6. **Protect Your Eyes:** Always wear the provided eye protection or goggles to safeguard your eyes from intense light exposure. Keep your eyes closed during the treatment.

7. **Position Properly:** Place the device or position yourself correctly to ensure that the light covers the intended treatment area. Follow recommended distances for optimal results.

8. **Be Consistent:** Develop a consistent treatment schedule and stick to it. Regular use, whether daily, a few times a week, or weekly, is essential for achieving desired outcomes.

9. **Monitor Progress:** Keep a record of your sessions and

observe how your body responds. Track any changes in your skin, pain levels, or other targeted conditions.

10. **Adjust as Needed:** If you're not experiencing the desired results, be open to adjusting your treatment plan. You can modify the duration, frequency, or even the device type as needed.

11. **Combine with Other Wellness Practices:** Red light therapy can complement other wellness practices. Maintain a balanced diet, engage in regular exercise, and prioritize good sleep for comprehensive well-being.

12. **Stay Hydrated:** Drink plenty of water before and after your

sessions, as red light therapy
may increase cellular activity
and hydration needs.

13. **Be Patient:** Understand that
red light therapy may take time
to yield noticeable results,
particularly for chronic
conditions. Be patient and
allow the therapy to work over
an extended period.

14. **Document Your Journey:**
Consider taking before-and-
after photos to visually track
your progress. This can be a
motivating way to witness the
changes over time.

15. **Share Experiences:** Engage
with online communities or
support groups dedicated to red
light therapy. Sharing
experiences and tips with others

can be both motivating and informative.

Red light therapy is a complementary approach to wellness and may not provide immediate or miraculous results. It is most effective when used as part of a holistic health plan. To maximize the benefits, it's essential to customize your approach to your individual goals and needs.

6.3 Tracking Your Progress

Tracking your progress in red light therapy is essential for understanding the effectiveness of your treatment and making necessary adjustments. Here's how to monitor and document your progress:

1. **Before-and-After Photos:**
   Take clear, well-lit photos of
   the area you are treating before
   you begin red light therapy.
   Continue taking photos at
   regular intervals, such as
   weekly or monthly, to
   document any changes in the
   condition you are targeting.
   Comparing these photos over
   time can provide visual
   evidence of your progress.

2. **Keep a Journal:** Maintain a
   journal or notebook dedicated
   to your red light therapy
   sessions. Record the date,
   duration of each session, any
   specific areas treated, and any
   observations or changes you
   notice. Note improvements or
   any adverse effects.

3. **Symptom and Pain Scales:** If you are using red light therapy to manage pain or a specific condition, consider using symptom or pain scales to quantify your experience. Rate the severity of your symptoms or pain on a scale from 1 to 10 before and after each session to gauge the changes.

4. **Measurable Metrics:** Some conditions, like skin health or hair growth, may have measurable metrics, such as skin texture, wrinkle depth, or hair thickness. Use tools or devices designed to measure these metrics and track changes over time.

5. **Subjective Assessments:** In addition to quantifiable measures, consider how you

subjectively feel. Document changes in how you feel physically, mentally, or emotionally. Do you feel more energetic, relaxed, or focused? These changes can be valuable indicators of the therapy's impact.

6. **Pain Diary:** If you are using red light therapy to manage chronic pain or inflammation, keep a pain diary. Note the frequency, duration, and intensity of your pain. Track any fluctuations and record how they correlate with your red light therapy sessions.

7. **Consult a Healthcare Professional:** If you have a medical condition that is being addressed with red light therapy, consult with a

healthcare professional for their input on tracking progress. They can offer guidance on what specific markers to monitor.

8. **Adherence to Schedule:** Monitor your adherence to the recommended schedule. Ensure that you are consistently following the treatment plan, as consistency is often key to success.

9. **Stay Informed:** Keep up-to-date with research and developments in red light therapy. New studies and findings may provide insights into the best ways to track and measure progress.

10. **Adjust as Needed:** Regularly review your progress tracking

data and consider making adjustments to your treatment plan as necessary. If you are not seeing the desired results, consult with a healthcare professional for guidance.

Progress may be gradual, and it may take time to see significant changes, especially for chronic conditions or those related to skin and beauty. Tracking your progress not only helps you understand the effectiveness of red light therapy but also provides motivation and helps you make informed decisions about your treatment plan.

6.4 Next Steps in Your Red-Light Therapy Journey

After you've initiated your red light therapy treatments and have made progress, it's important to consider what steps to take next. Here are some suggestions for the next steps in your red light therapy journey:

1. **Assess Your Progress:** Regularly evaluate your progress based on the tracking methods you've been using, whether it's photos, journals, pain scales, or other measurements. This will help you determine whether you're achieving your goals and whether any adjustments are needed.

2. **Consult a Healthcare Professional:** If you've been using red light therapy to address a specific medical condition, consult with a healthcare professional to discuss your progress. They can provide guidance on whether to continue, modify, or discontinue treatment based on your outcomes.

3. **Refine Your Treatment Plan:** Based on your assessment and any advice from a healthcare professional, you can refine your treatment plan. This may involve altering the frequency, duration, or areas of treatment.

4. **Explore New Goals:** If you've achieved your initial goals, consider whether there are additional health or wellness

objectives you'd like to target
with red light therapy. It's a
versatile tool with potential
applications beyond your initial
goals.

5. **Consider Combination
   Therapies:** Explore the
   potential benefits of combining
   red light therapy with other
   wellness practices, such as diet,
   exercise, or complementary
   therapies. A holistic approach
   to health often yields the best
   results.

6. **Stay Informed:** Continue to
   educate yourself about red light
   therapy by staying informed
   about the latest research and
   developments in the field. New
   studies may offer insights into
   novel applications or best
   practices.

7. **Share Your Experience:** If you've had positive results with red light therapy, consider sharing your experience with others who may benefit. You can provide valuable insights and encouragement to those who are just starting their journey.

8. **Stay Committed:** To maintain and build upon your progress, it's essential to stay committed to your red light therapy routine. Consistency is often a key factor in achieving long-term benefits.

9. **Maintain Safety:** As you continue your red light therapy journey, it's important to prioritize safety. Follow safety guidelines and use the therapy

responsibly to avoid adverse effects.

10. **Keep an Open Mind:** Red light therapy is a dynamic field with ongoing research and discoveries. Be open to trying new approaches or devices that may offer improvements or more tailored solutions.

11. **Consult Device Manufacturers:** If you're using a specific red light therapy device, reach out to the manufacturer for guidance, support, or any questions you may have.

Red light therapy journey is a dynamic process that can evolve as your health and wellness needs change. Regular assessment, professional guidance, and staying informed are essential to making the most of this therapeutic approach.

www.ingramcontent.com/pod-product-compliance
Lightning Source LLC
Chambersburg PA
CBHW050842260726
48660CB00006B/2401